I0706627

Survival Medicine Guide:

86 Most Effective Remedies And Best

Recipes To Cure Children With Healing

Herbss

Disclaimer: All photos used in this book, including the cover photo were made available under a Attribution-Non Commercial-Share Alike 2.0 Generic and sourced from Flickr

Table of content:

Book 1

Survival Medicine: 30 Best Essential Oils, Healing Herbs And Salves For Excellent Health + 22 Effective Natural Remedies For The Treatment Of Diseases... **5**

Introduction.. 6

Chapter 1. Aromatherapy as Survival Medicine 11

Chapter 2. Herbs as Survival Medicine. 15

Chapter 3. Soothing Survival Salves... 23

Chapter 4. Diseases and there remedies 28

Conclusion 47

Book 2

Essential Oils for Kids: 34 DIY Natural Toxic-Free Recipes For Your Children's Health **50**

Introduction..51

Chapter 1 - Aromatherapy for Kids 101 52

Chapter 2 - Essential Oil List... 60

Chapter 3 - The Immune System.. 64

Chapter 4 - Dry Skin 71

Chapter 5 - Homework and Concentration 76

Chapter 6 - Bedtime and Nervousness.. 80

Chapter 7 - Bath Time... 82

Chapter 8 - Tips and Tricks 86

Conclusion 87

SURVIVAL MEDICINE

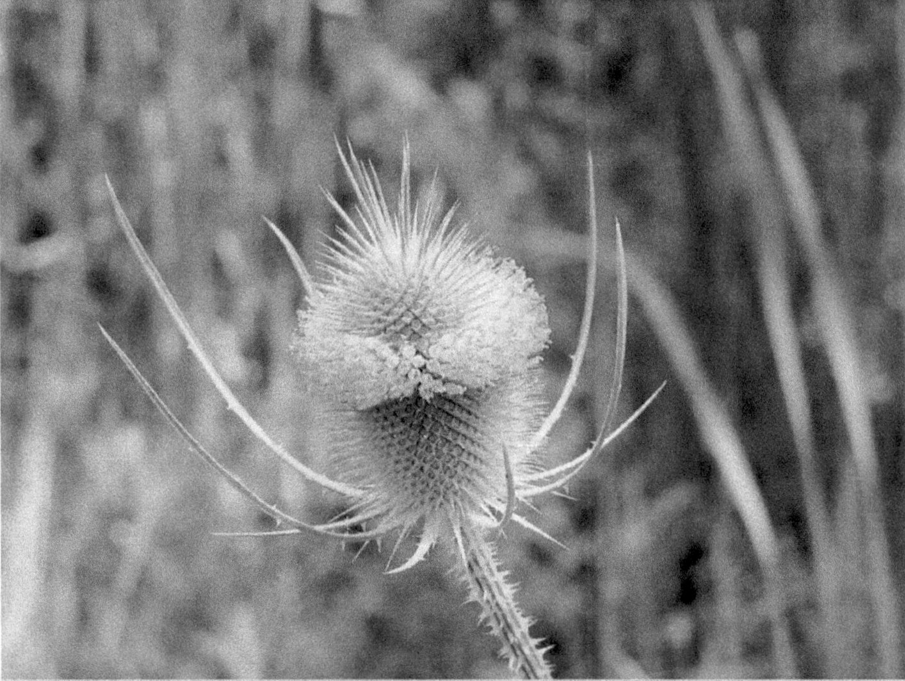

30 Best Essential Oils, Healing Herbs
And Salves For Excellent Health
+ 22 Effective Natural
Remedies For The Treatment Of Diseases

CRYSTAL WILKINS

Survival Medicine:

30 Best Essential Oils, Healing Herbs And Salves For Excellent Health + 22 Effective Natural Remedies For The Treatment Of Diseases

Introduction.

Health is intrinsically linked with everything we do. If you can keep yourself in the right physical state, you will be much better predisposed to be in the right mental state. So it is that the basics of our health are the basis of happiness itself. If you want to be healthy both mind and body in order to survive an emergency, let's get down to the basics of health!

Preparing for the unpredictable is not an oxymoron it is simply being proactive in a troubled world. And in any crisis situation our health should be of number one concern to us.

One of the most important things before picking the right survival medicine is to have the basic knowledge about its usage. It is really important that you identify herbs correctly. We have provided photographs of most of these herbs and have added additional information about their appearance so that you can hand-pick the natural herbs of your choice.

After when you have identified the natural products that can help you survive, the second most important factor is regarding their correct usage. We have listed the most appropriate way to use these herbs and how they can help you in various ways. A proper listing of their benefits has been provided so that you can figure out how and when to use these herbs correctly.

A single herb can be of numerous usages and you should certainly keep a few of them with you when you move, as an unforeseen disaster might come unannounced. A wide range of natural herbs have been discussed in the guide – from edible products to antiseptic ones, anti-inflammatory herbs to plants that can help in skin treatment, and more.

Health is intrinsically linked with everything we do. If you can keep yourself in the right physical state, you will be much better predisposed to be in the right mental state. So it is that the basics of our health are the basis of happiness itself. If you want to be healthy both mind and body in order to survive an emergency, let's get down to the basics of Survival Medicine!

First Aid is not only for lifesaving purposes, it is also an invaluable tool for managing everyday injuries and illnesses that can occur in your home or any other environment. Interestingly, the numbers of injuries that take place in the home are staggering when compared to those that occur in other places.

Think of the times you may have tripped and fallen over the cat, burnt yourself cooking, struck your thumb with a hammer during home maintenance, or simply spent too much time out in the sun mowing your lawn. And if you have children, the numbers of at home injuries increase dramatically!

Knowing the basics of first aid is also essential if you plan on doing any outdoor excursions, particularly in the wilderness or out on the water. There, you can face a lot of hidden dangers that don't exist in your urban neighborhood, and it is much harder to dash to the emergency room or get paramedic help. In those types of situations, survival is down to you.

Being prepared for any scenario can increase your chances of survival. This is also true of natural disasters, as these can strike at any time without any warning. Tornados, hurricanes, earthquakes, are all extreme forces of nature, and loss of life is a very real possibility, so if you know first aid, not only can you help yourself and your family, but also you're neighbors, and the greater community. Your skills would be invaluable in these types of situations. But first, you need to know how to assess a situation.

Steps to Properly Assess the Situation

Step 1: Minimize Risk

The number one priority in any emergency situation is to first ensure that you as the rescuer are not in any danger. Look around the area and check that whatever caused the injury is no longer a threat. Do not put yourself at risk, or you too could become a victim, which then leaves nobody to assist.

Step 2: Primary Assessment

This is where you check the airway, breathing and circulation of the victim. Note whether or not the victim is breathing, and how they are breathing. You may need to explore the mouth with your fingers to see if there is an obstruction of the airway.

Next, check the circulation by feeling for a pulse either on the neck, the inside of the wrist, or if necessary the groin.

The next part of the assessment is to check whether or not there is an injury to the spinal cord. If this type of injury is suspected, the person should not be moved, and the neck must be supported at all times.

Also note the temperature of the environment, particularly if it is very hot or very cold, as this could have a huge impact on the victim. If they can't be moved, cover them with something to keep them warm, or create a shield from the heat using whatever is nearby and available.

Step 3: Secondary Assessment

Once you have ascertained the victim is breathing and has a pulse, the next step in the assessment process is to determine whether or not there are injuries. This could involve speaking to the victim if they are conscious and asking where they are feeling any pain. If the victim is unconscious, you will need to check for injuries by gently feeling and looking at the body from the head to the toes.

At this point you will also be checking for any discoloration, such as blueness or pale color of the face which may indicate an internal issue such as shock.

First Aid Basics

DRSABCD

DRSABCD is a formula that is taught to anyone learning first aid. This acronym is important to remember, as it will help you follow the correct procedures when faced with an emergency medical situation. The acronym stands for:

D – Danger

Check that there is no further risk or danger to yourself first, then the others around you including the injured or sick person.

R – Response

Note whether or not the person is conscious or responds to your voice or touch.

S – Send for Help

If possible, call emergency services, or if necessary, send someone to get help.

A – Airway

Check the airway and make sure it is clear of any obstruction.

B – Breathing

Look to see if the chest is moving up and down as it would during breathing. Alternatively, listen to their breath sounds near the mouth or nose.

C – Cardiopulmonary Resuscitation (CPR)

If the victim is not breathing and is unconscious, begin CPR.

D – Defibrillate

If a defibrillation device is available, and the situation requires it, use it.

Chapter 1. Aromatherapy as Survival Medicine

Aromatherapy is an ancient practice with powerful results for modern survival medicine. Just take a look at the following examples and how they can greatly enrich your life—no matter the situation.

Frankincense Oil

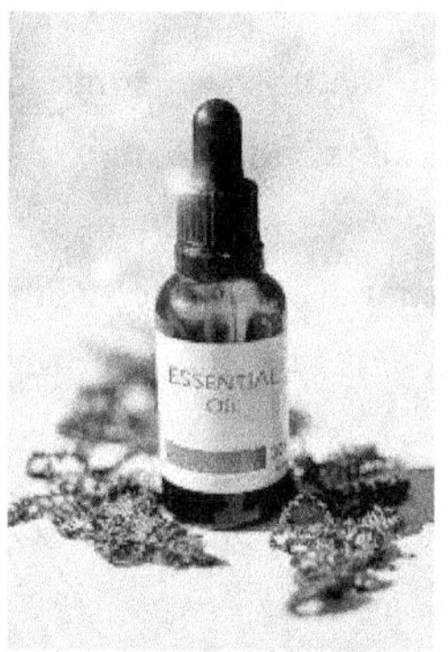

Frankincense has a long history of use. It was prized in ancient times both for its alluring aroma and for its healing properties. Just rub this essential oil into the skin and the healing properties of this herb will work to holistically treat your entire body. It boosts the immune system and cleanses at the same time.

In order to administer Frankincense Oil, either breathe in the aroma from a fresh bottle of essential oil or place a few drops in an incense burner and let the aroma fill the entire room, so that you can benefit from the treatment gradually as you go about your day.

Jasmine Oil

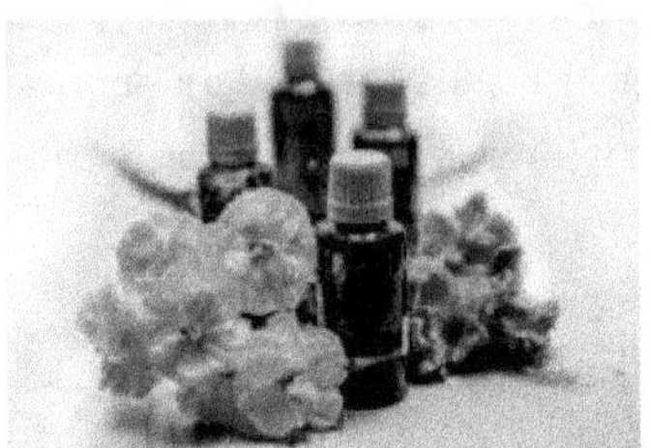

Jasmine has quite a lovely aroma and most that have breathed it in will agree to how refreshing it can be. And when you concentrate the oil of jasmine down to its most powerful form for aroma therapy the effects can be downright life changing. This essential oil has been known to boost memory and overall mental focus for those that use it. Just breathe in a few drops of this stuff and you will know the true meaning of aromatherapy for survival medicine.

Peppermint Oil

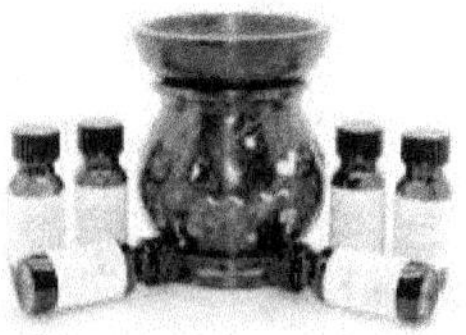

This refreshing blast of peppermint will help to calm your nerves and maybe even boost your metabolism! Peppermint is also known to open up the breathing passages so if you are having any trouble with congestion of shortness of breath, you may want to seriously give peppermint a try. As an asthma sufferer myself I can attest to the healing power of peppermint. Just a few whiffs of this stuff and I am all better. So be sure to keep some of this wondrous healing herb on hand for your own survival medicine.

Coriander Oil

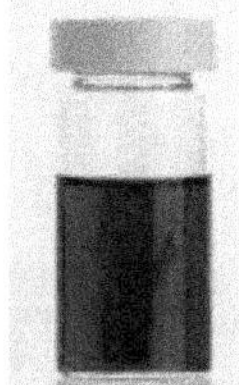

I was first exposed to coriander oil as something to cook with. But little did I know that coriander oil is also great for aromatherapy. Just by breathing in the aroma of this oil you will be able to greatly increase the blood supply of your cardiovascular system. This extra burst of blood flow will actually help your body to relax considerably. So if you feel like may need a break, just breathe in some coriander oil.

Grapefruit Oil

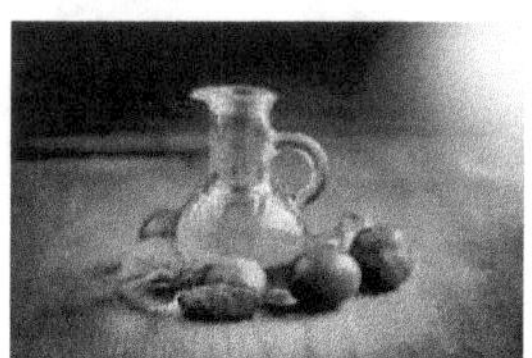

The powerful aromatherapy provided by grapefruit oil can work to really get you going in the morning! This essential oil when breathed in directly will allow for your body to get that extra boost it needs to get through the day. Regular regimens of breathing in this oil could also greatly improve your mental clarity and recall of events. So yes, I would advise, if you need survival medicine, then you need to give some grapefruit oil a try!

Neola Oil

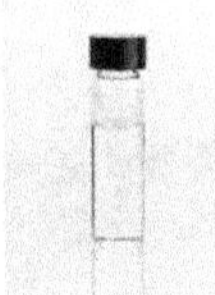

The effect of this essential oil when breathed into the body through a regular routine of aromatherapy is almost immediate. As soon as you breathe it in you will begin to feel your heart beat just a little bit slower. And after your treatment progresses your whole body will soon be relaxed! Neola oil is highly recommended!

Cyprus Oil

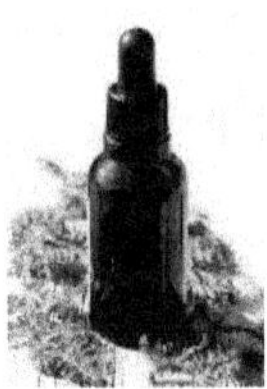

You may have noticed the scent of cypress in many cars you have been driven in since Cyprus is the number one scent in car air fresheners. You may have had the privilege of sitting under a tree shaped car air freshener and breathed in that tree-like scent. Well this essential oil is also quite effective as a form of aromatic treatment for a wide range of illnesses and discomforts.

Most notably this aromatic oil is great for giving those who breathe it in a refreshing calm and an increase in overall energy. So if you need a bit of a boost at any time during yo9ur day you should just take some time to stop and smell the Cyprus!

Chapter 2. Herbs as Survival Medicine.

Milk Thistle

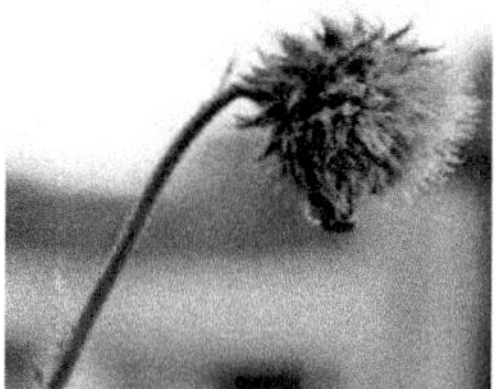

This herb is another great item to pack in your medicine chest. With its ability to reduce inflammation, this herb has been known to have some rather amazing results. Milk thistle serves to boost liver function and in some instances has even been seen to reverse the effects of cirrhosis. If you have any inflammation whatsoever, simply apply some Milk Thistle directly to the area afflicted and you will see results.

Red Clover

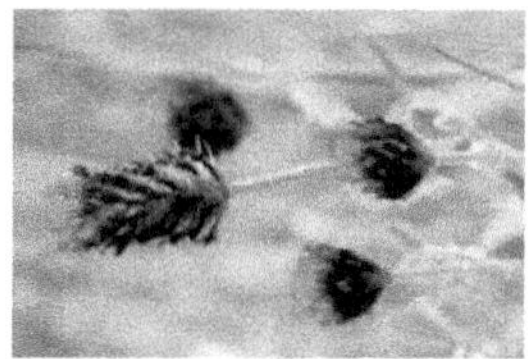

Red Clover is a powerful herbal antibiotic that can greatly boost the immune system. This herb has even been known to increase the red blood cell count in those that use it. Interestingly enough, Red Clover is also a natural anticoagulant and can loosen up blood clots in rather rapid fashion. This in turn provides a general boost in health no matter what you may be facing.

Yarrow

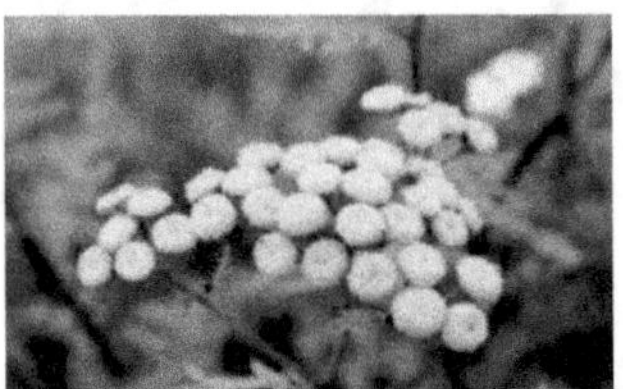

Yarrow is an herb that has been used for centuries; and with good reason. This herb can get to work on inflammation and congestion in the human body, almost immediately. This herbal antibiotic also works well against injuries, and as soon as it is applied to an injured site, it gets to work cleansing the injury and promoting the formation for blood platelets for a quick and effective healing.

Gauche

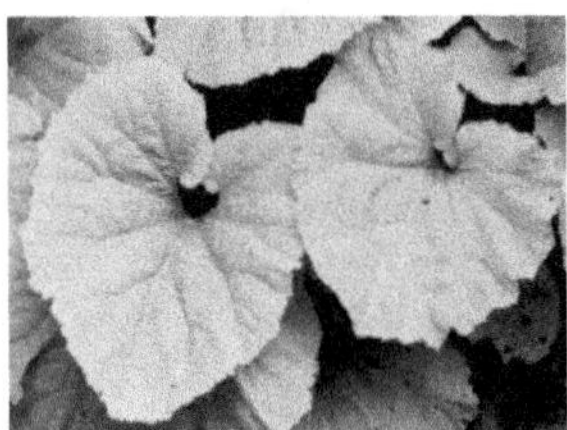

This herb is a great antibiotic fighter and its best work is done to reduce inflammation and boost the immune system. Just apply a small amount of this herbal antibiotic to the skin and you will be able to enhance your body's ability to stand up to and survive all manner of airborne illnesses. Give this herbal Gauche Antibiotic a try!

Ginkgo

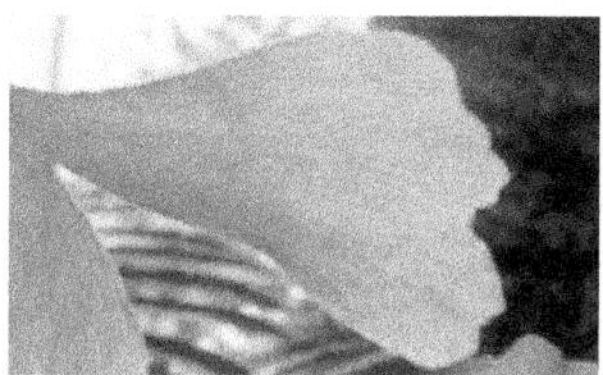

Ginkgo is a powerful and useful allergy fighter and works to reduce inflammation. This herb is also great when it comes to improving the flow of oxygen to the brain. It is for this reason that so many take Ginkgo to boost their memory and concentration. So if you are feeling at all slow and sluggish in the morning—or any other time for that matter—a good dose of Ginkgo tea could really do you some good! This tea can be made through either boiling powdered Ginkgo or raw Ginkgo leaves.

Anise

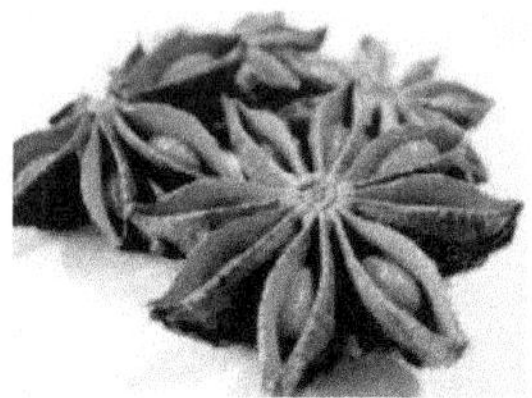

This herb works out just great as an herbal antibiotic, killing most bacteria right on the spot. This herbal antibiotic also works on the urinary system, helping to clear up any incontinence that someone may be facing, and putting the whole body into a kind of detox, almost immediately. One of the best ways to administer this healing herb is to boil it into a nice and tasty tea. So drink up folks because this Herbal Anise is on me!

Chervil

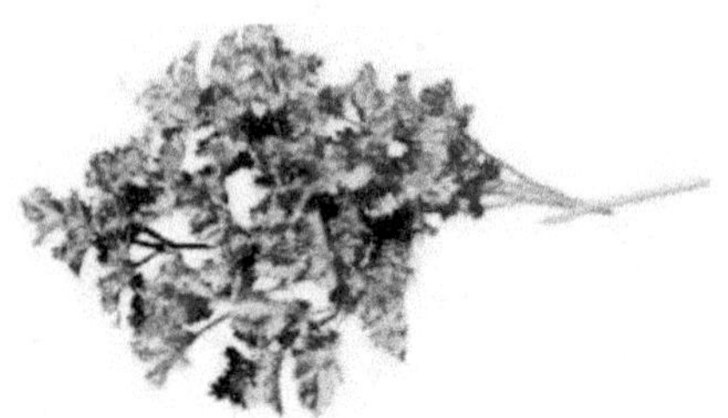

Chervil has a real proven ability when it comes to killing bacteria, getting rid of headaches and calming upset stomachs. It is the latter from which many a camper has benefited. It is common practice for many survivalists to simply pop a leaf of chervil in their mouth and chew in order to relieve their upset stomach. I have tried this myself and can say that it really does wonders.

Cloves

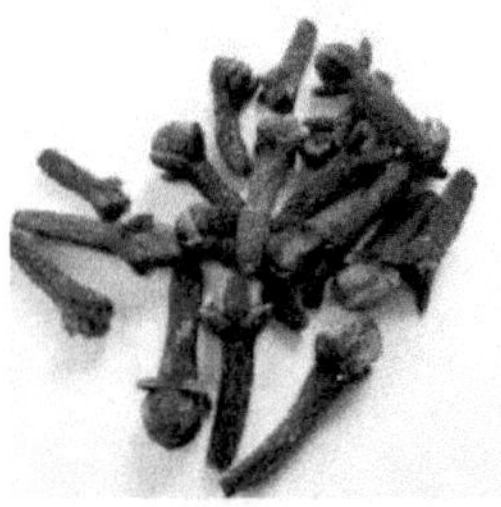

In a similar fashion to chervil, cloves have been placed directly into the mouth of many dental patients in order to kill bacteria and curb inflammatory agents. This herb also works as a mild form of pain reliever and can be used to successfully numb up a bad toothache if needed.

Sage

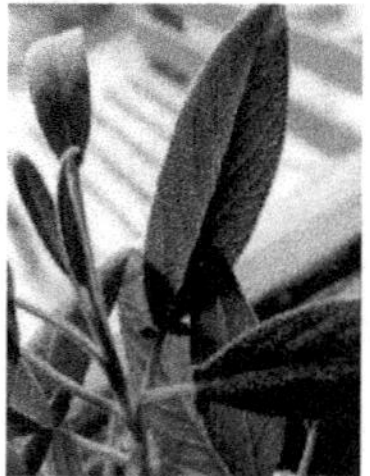

This medicinal herb takes survival medicine to a whole new live in the way that it can successfully reduce all manner of pain and kill bacterial infections on the spot. If you have fallen and sustained an injury, just a very small application of this healing herb will work to alleviate any pain that you may feel. Another great benefit of herbal sage is its ability to treat asthma. I have suffered with asthma most of my life myself, and applications of this herb have helped to improve my own breathing considerably when I have tried it.

Valerian

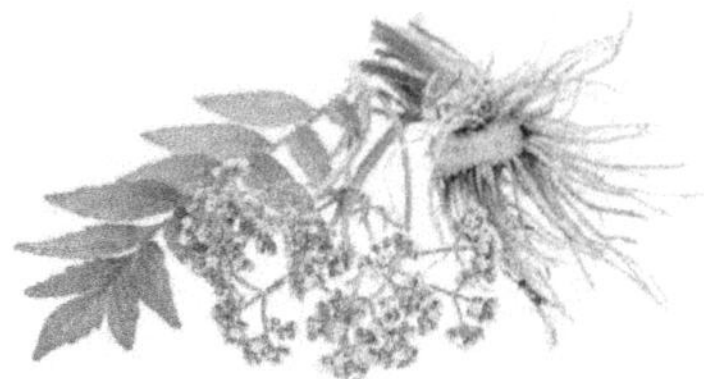

Valerian is also another very popular nighttime home remedies to deal with your anxiety. It contains some elements of mild tranquilizing properties that will almost guarantee you and will get you a good night sleep. However, without all dreaded and the weird hangover feeling early in the morning that you may sometimes have to get with some other pharmaceuticals.

Passionflower

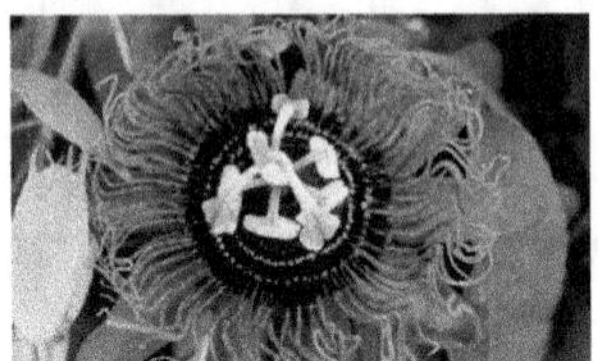

Passionflower is also referred to as folk for a natural remedy and anxiety, insomnia and panic attacks. Passionflower has been shown in many studies to treat anxiety is a very remarkably well.

One study has found it has to be as effective as benzodiazepine drugs, but the only difference is without the drowsiness. Passionflower may also help you to feel an emotionally balanced and exceptionally beneficial way.

Nonetheless, if you suffer from exaggerated emotions then this is by far one of the most efficient home remedies to deal with anxiety, and it needs to be part of your daily regimen.

Lemon Balm

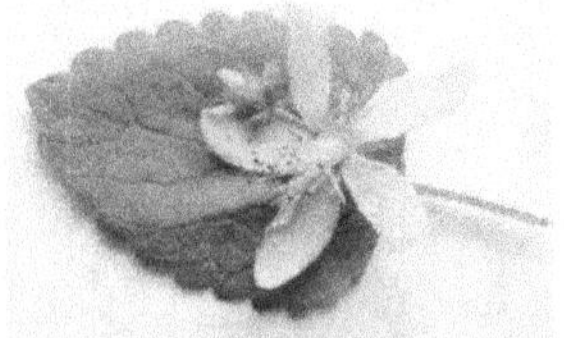

Lemon Balm also is known as 'Melissa officinalis' which is one herbal supplement and tea to treat anxiety and calm your nerves.

Some studies suggested that the use of lemon balm can decrease insomnia, anxiety, hyper excitation and fatigue.

A lemon balm extract which should be taken 300mg at breakfast and 300mg at dinner too which may help reduced insomnia mainly due to a decrease in nervousness and also to decreased agitation, guilt, hyper excitation and fatigue too.

California poppy

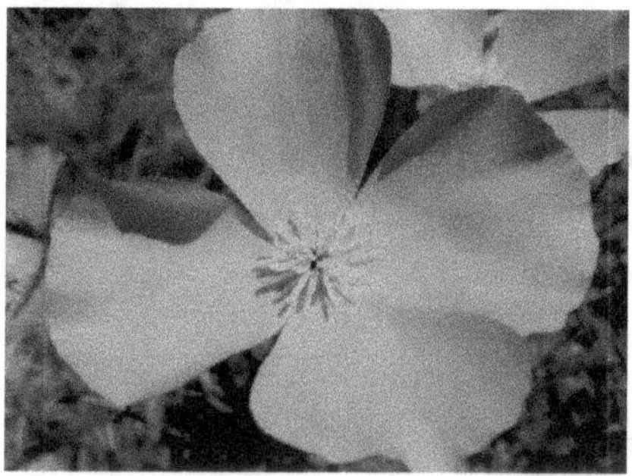

California poppy also called Eschscholtzia californica, which is a tension-relieving, anti-anxiety, sedative, and antispasmodic herb. California poppy also helps with sleeplessness and quells a headache as well as muscular spasm from stress. Some gentle and non-addictive actions are much safer for children and the elderly.

Wild Lettuce

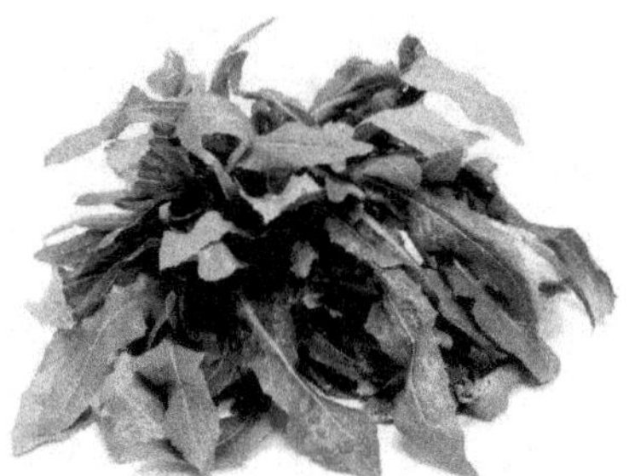

Wild Lettuce is of the species of lactic vireos, which is a mild tranquilizer that may be used for calming a nervous or overactive nervous system. It is very suitable for anxious children or even adolescents. It majorly helps with insomnia. It is also a general pain reliever and antispasmodic that can primarily be used for short coughs.

Rosemary

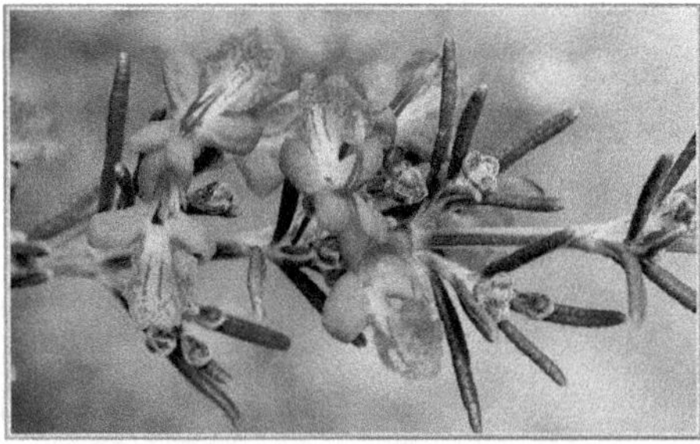

The herb that makes chicken sing and soups taste wonderful helps treat headaches, nervous tension, a nervous stomach, cleanse the face, and can even help to stimulate hair growth. Great in teas, oils, and soaks.

Chapter 3. Soothing Survival Salves

Here are a few healing salves that will help you survive just about anything that comes your way!

Almond Lip Salve

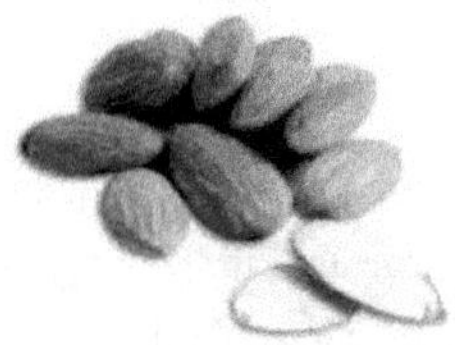

This healing salve is a natural way to cure dry lips. If you have repeatedly dry and cracking lips you can greatly benefit by even the smallest of applications of this herbal lip balm. This lip balm is almost odorless and has just a slightly sweet taste that will not interfere with eating or anything else you do throughout the course of a day.

Coconut Salve

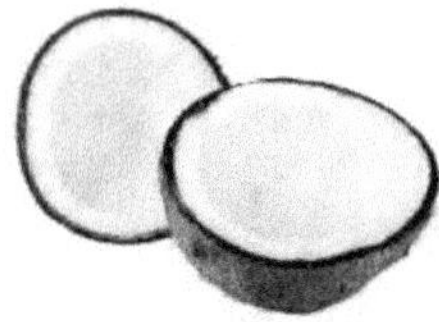

Coconut salves are always classy and soothing. This salve is no exception. Made out of concentrated coconut oil, just a little dab will do you! Place this coconut salve on your lips, feet, arms, or any other part of your being that could use just a little bit of soothing!

Lemon Balm Salve

Lemon Balm is perhaps one of the most popular salves that you could ever use. These salves are great for chapped lips and even better for rough hands. You can also use this salve as an herbal antibiotic since lemon naturally kills all germs and bacteria on contact. Lemon balm salve is also great for the face and even small applications of it can help can clear up complexions and even treat wrinkling of the skin.

Cat's Claw Salve

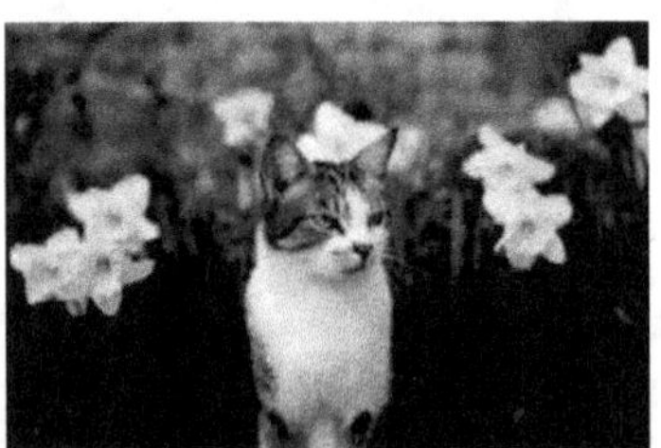

This healing salve is a great immune booster and can even help promote the production of white blood cells when regularly applied to the skin. Simply put; external viruses, bacteria, and other germs don't stand a chance when cat's claw is applied!

Burdock Root

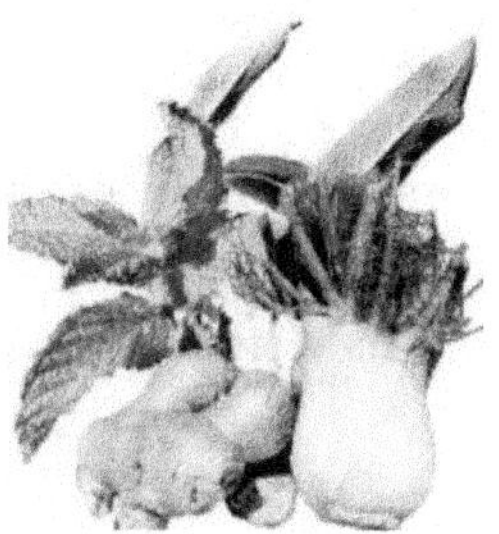

If you are suffering from arthritis, the inflammation fighting power of a little Burdock Root could be just what the doctor ordered for you. Just a brief application of this healing salve and your arthritis will be long behind you. Be sure to pack this herbal healing salve in your bag as part of your survival medicine arsenal.

Aloe Vera

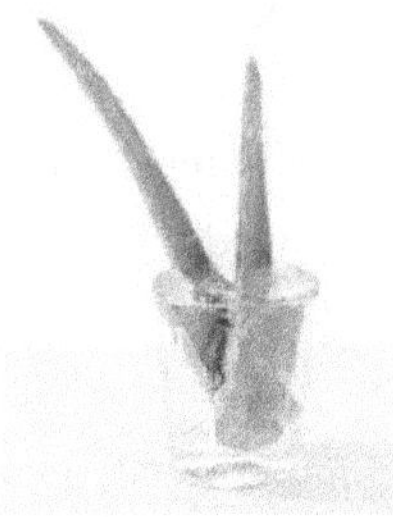

Burns have met their match with Aloe Vera. This healing salve sooths even as it protects. As soon as you apply Aloe Vera to a burn on the skin you will feel the soothing relief that this herb can provide. Burns by their nature—as well as damaging tissue structure—take all of the moisture out of the injury.

But an application of Aloe Vera will put that moisture back in. So don't hesitate to bring yourself some Aloe Vera folks!

The best way to pack it is in a tube, but *if you can hack it*, you can make some of your own. All you have to do is take the Aloe Vera leaf, split it open and then scoop the gel out. Either way you will have a powerful and soothing herbal healing salve on your hands.

Dandelion

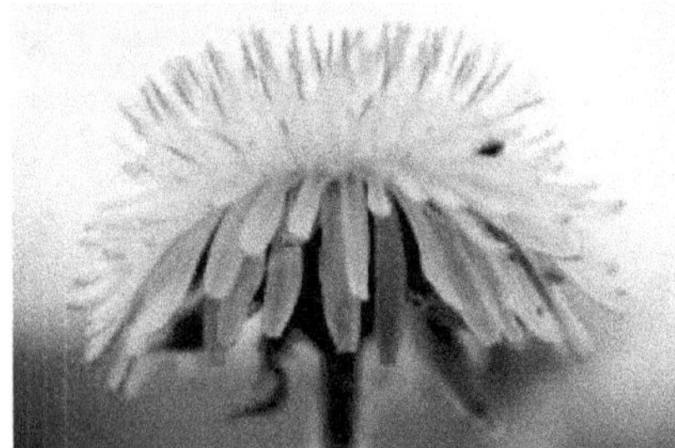

Dandelions are quite prolific, you see than sprouting up in yards, parking lots and businesses all across the country. The bane of lawnmowers and weed whackers everywhere—these little yellow guys really do get around.

And this healing salve once applied can do wonders for everything from allergies to immune system protection. Improving the production of platelets in the blood, this healing salve has been shown to even improve the lives of cancer patients. So this is definitely a survival medicine tat could be of some great use for you.

Ashwagandha

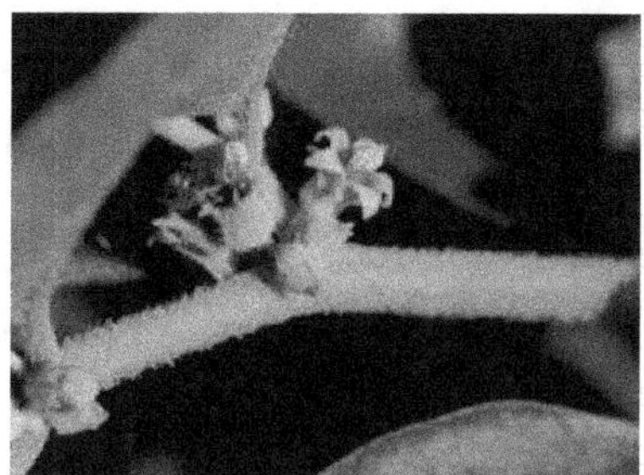

This healing salve has been with us for quite some time, and known as an "adaptogen" it can work to adapt to just about any situation that is thrown at it. Ashwagandha can help with everything from inflammation, to boosting immune health, to healing injuries from cuts, scrapes, and burns. All of this makes for some great soothing survival salves!

Chapter 4. Diseases and there remedies

Heartburn

This is an over production of stomach acids to different degrees. Many antacids on the market can make this worse instead of better, leading to a complete dependence to the medication.

Here are some simple things you can do to help when it flares up:

• Parsley helps to curve heartburn. Chewing on a sprig will release the juice and stem the acid flow.

• Peppermint tea will help cool the burn.

Heartburn Tea

1 tsp Peppermint
(cools the core)
1 tsp Chamomile Flowers
1 tsp Lemon Balm leaves cut
(helps curve acid)
Drink cold

Marshmallow and Chamomile syrup

1 Ounce Marshmallow Root
(helps to absorb acids)
1 Ounce Chamomile Flowers
(calms the stomach)
2 Ounces Raw Honey
1 Tbsp every four to six hours.

Upset Stomach

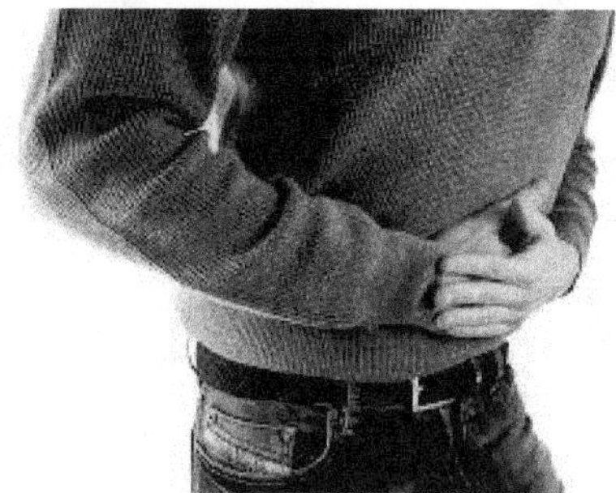

This can be as small as an upset stomach to nausea and vomiting. Here are couple of things you can try:

• Chewing on a clove and swallowing the juice will alleviate nausea

• Putting a small amount of Allspice powder under your tongue will do the same.

Calming Tummy Tea

1 tsp Chamomile Flowers
1 tsp Peppermint leaves
1 tsp Fennel Seeds
(soothes the stomach)

Calming Tummy Syrup

1/2 ounce Peppermint Leaves
1/2 ounce Fennel Seeds
1/2 ounce Anise Seeds
1/2 ounce Lavender flowers
2 ounces raw honey

Nervous System

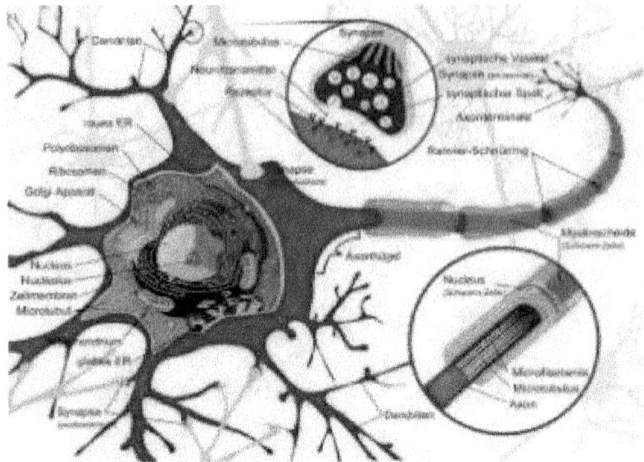

Made of our brain, eyes, spinal cord, and millions of synapses that fire off in order to deliver information to the brain the nervous system is truly a marvel, and many biologist have yet to unlock all its mysteries, but there are some ailments that are prevalent today which herbs to can help stem, if not help cure.

Alzheimer's Disease

Given a name in the late 80's this disease causes dementia in a patient, often reverting them back to child-like behavior and erasing memories of past experiences and even loved ones. There have been many reports of patients wandering off or family members getting in a car and driving only to not realize where they are.

Gingko Biloba has been tested, and in double blind studies has shown it can reverse early stages of Alzheimer's and lessen the severity of later stages.

Senility

This is quite different from dementia. Instead of wandering off or losing memories, it begins to present itself as being absent-minded and not able to recall things right away. This is simply due to the fact we need more B vitamins as we get older to help our brain function at the levels we are used to and for our nervous systems to function as they should.

Tea for concentration

1 tsp Peppermint leaves
1 tsp Gingko Bilboa
1 tsp Kelp (for B vitamins)

Extract for concentration

1 ounce Peppermint
1 ounce Kelp
1 ounce Gingko Biloba
1 ounce Gotu Kola
(Does the same thing as Gingko)

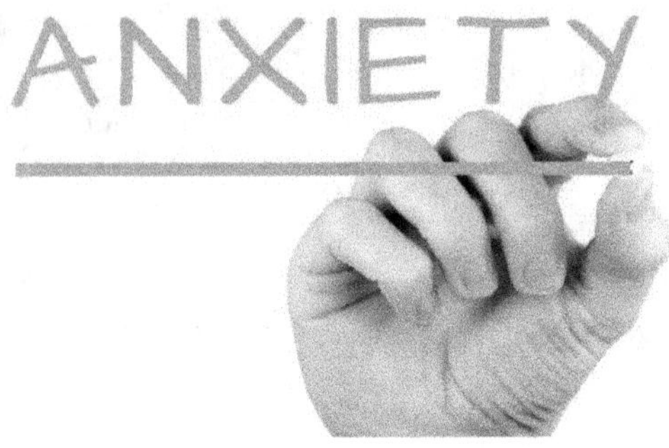

Anxiety can be debilitating. It can completely cripple someone leaving them unable to function. Here are couple of remedies that can help.

Nerve Tea

1 tsp Chamomile Flowers
1 tsp Catnip leaves
1 tsp Lavender Flowers

Herbal Bath

1/2 Ounce Lavender Flowers
1/2 Ounce Chamomile Flowers

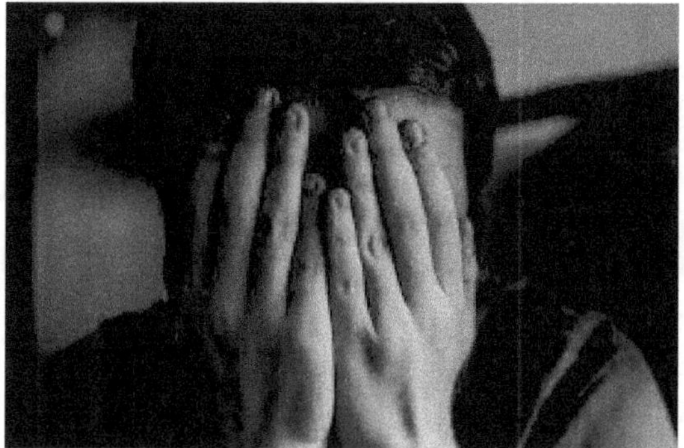

Many people suffer from depression. It can take hours out of the day from your life by making you feel lethargic, and uninterested in everyday things. Just keep in mind, if you are bi-polar, you will have seek further advice from a licensed physician. The same goes for depression caused by chemical imbalances.

Saint John's Wort is the best herb to take for depression provided you are not already taking anti-depression medication.

Arthritis

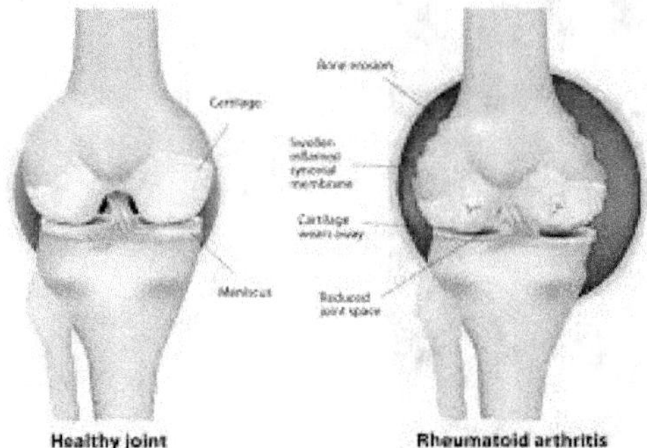

This is a condition that attacks the joints and causes swelling, pain, and loss of movement/mobility. There are dietary restrictions to help prevent the swelling:

• Avoid the nightshade vegetables like tomatoes, potatoes, eggplant, and peppers.

• Keeping a diary of what you eat and how your arthritis reacts to what you eat can add to that list of foods to avoid.

These are skin conditions that are visible on the skin and can range from rashes that are cracked and bleeding to scale-like rashes that weep. Even though there are prescription medications that claim to bring these conditions under control, but they do it by suppressing the immune system, which can expose you to more serious diseases.

There are two ways to start being proactive when it comes to controlling these conditions:

• Get an allergy test. It have been proven, in some cases, these are allergic reactions to either environmental factors or food you eat.

• Manage your stress. This is easier said than done, but learning how to relieve and control stress will work wonders for controlling and, in some cases, relieve the condition altogether.

Bruise Salve

1 Cup of Sweet Almond oil (or Apricot Kernel oil if you're allergic to tree nuts)
1/8 Cup Beeswax
1 Tbsp *Arnica flowers*
(Really good for bruises)
1 Tbsp *Lavender Flowers*
(Good for Swelling)
(You can substitute Chamomile here)
1 Tbsp *Echinacea*
(Speeds healing)

Bruise poultice

2 Tbsp Arnica Flowers
Echinacea Tea

Joint Muscle Rub

6 Ounces of Sweet Almond Oil
2 Ounces of Olive Oil
2 Tbsp Juniper Berries
(Swelling and joint pain)
2 Tbsp Devil's Claw
(Joint pain and ligaments)
1 Tbsp Cinnamon
(Swelling and heating effect)
2 Tbsp Peppermint Leaves
(Cooling effect and anti-inflammatory)

Joint Herbal Bath

1/2 Ounce of Juniper Berries
1/2 Ounce of Lavender or Chamomile Flowers

Eczema Ointment

2 Tbsp Kelp (Smooths the skin)
2 Tbsp Chamomile Flowers (helps smooth skin)
2 Tbsp Echinacea
2 Tbsp Avocado Butter (for extra moisture)

Psoriasis Rub

1/4 Cup Shea Butter

1/4 Cup Avocado Butter

(Both are excellent to toning and softening the skin and adding moisture)

2 Tbsp Lavender flowers

2 Tbsp Rose Petals

2 Tbsp Peppermint Leaves

1/4 ounce Aloe leaf

- Place the butters in a crock pot
- Add the herbs and steep overnight
- Strain out the herbs and place in a container with a tight lid.
- Let it cool before completely tightening the lid.
- Rub into the patches.

The Circulatory System

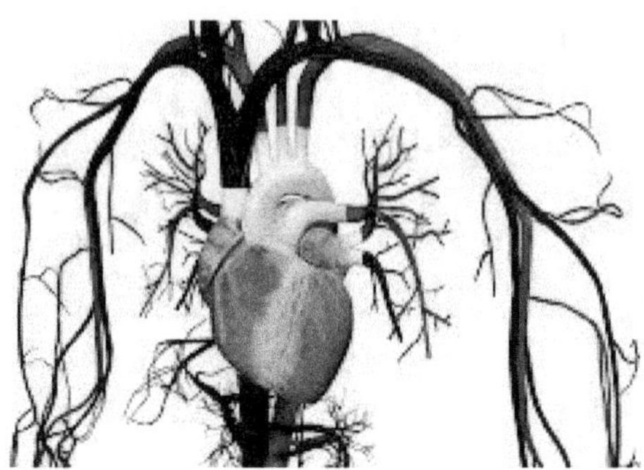

Your heart and blood vessels are the carriers of the oxygen that leaves you lungs. They also help you convey vitamins, minerals, and amino acids to your muscles. When your blood vessels start to clog, you can experience shortness of breath, low energy, and put your heart at risk because it's trying to work harder to get the blood to where it needs to go.

Heart disease and hypertension are two of the most prominent problems in our society. Taking care of your heart is very important for a healthy life.

Hypertension

Simply put this is very high blood pressure on a regular/daily basis. Left untreated, it can lead to heart attack and stroke.

As the skin condition above, relieving and learning how to manage stress can help lower blood pressure.

Changes in diet can do this as well. Even walking three times a week for at least twenty minutes can reduce your blood pressure. Here are a couple of recipes that can help without interacting with any medications you may be taking.

For a Weak Heart

Some people are born with congenital heart disease or a weak heart. This leads to them tiring easily and being short of breath.

Infusion for weak valves

1 tsp hawthorn berries crushed
(Highly recommended for a weak heart)
1 tsp night blooming cereus
(for valve malfunctions)
1 tsp catnip
(nervine)
Makes 1 therapeutic strength cup or 3 6-ounce regular strength cups.

Post-op Heart Attack Decoction

1 tsp hawthorn berries
1 tsp Dan Sheng Root
(Helps speed healing from heart operations)
1 tsp Lemon Zest (for flavor)
1 tsp Lavender flowers
(reduces swelling)

Hypertension

Just cooking with Basil and Cardamom can help to reduce your blood pressure. You can find these at any grocery store. Cooking with flaxseed is another way to help reduce your blood pressure.

Tea for Hypertension

Ginger tea is excellent for hypertension but if you can't handle the bite you can add Lavender and a little raw orange juice.

Blood Builders

These two recipes are to help strengthen blood vessels and for those who have low iron in their blood.

Iron Tea

1 tsp Red Raspberry leaves
1 tsp Red Clover flowers cut
1 tsp Butcher's Broom

Varicose Vein Bath

1/2 ounce Butcher's Broom
1/2 ounce Burdock Root

Migraines

There are headaches that can be a nuisance and there are migraines that can make chunks of your absolutely miserable with a spike is driven through your head. Thought they are still trying to figure out all the root causes of migraines there are few things you can do to help stave some of them off:

- Log smells, foods and other things that can trigger a migraine.
- High stress can also cause migraines.

You can help relieve stress by meditation, and listening to soothing music when you come home from a busy day.

Migraine Tea

1 tsp Feverfew
1 tsp Peppermint

The Glandular System

This is the system that can regulate everything from the metabolism to you hormones and everything in between. Even though the liver is generally considered part of the digestive system, I have put it here because of it's filtering abilities and how it aids the pancreas in regulating blood sugar levels.

Diabetes

This is a well-known disease which involves the pancreas. Insulin is created by the pancreas to regulate blood sugar, but when starts to malfunction, it can produce less and less, leading to higher levels of glucose in the blood.

This can cause dizziness and fainting spells, mood swings, and in more severe cases diabetic comas.

Nopal can help regulate glucose levels, and Stevia, a natural sweetener that is 10x sweeter than sugar, can as well.

Blood Sugar Tea

1 tsp Juniper Berries
1 tsp Ginger
1 tsp Billberry

Blood sugar Capsules

Equal parts of the following herbs in powder form:

Juniper berries
Nopal
Billberry
Stevia

It is recommended that you constantly check your blood sugar level if you are already on medication for this to make sure you are not lowering your glucose levels to dangerous numbers.

Liver/ Gall Bladder

The Liver

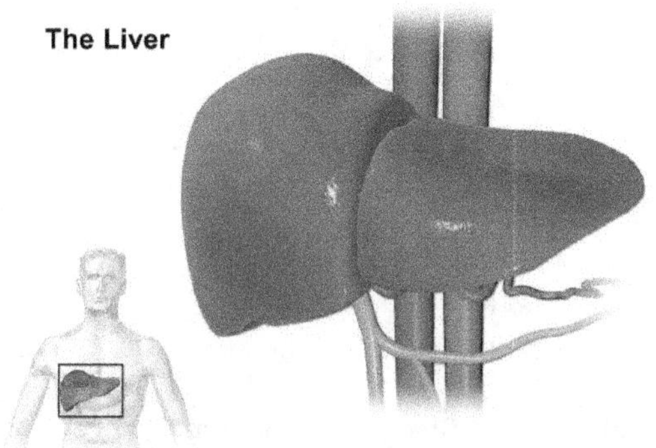

Your liver and gall bladder take the brunt of the abuse when it comes to filtering out any toxins in your system. From fats to alcohol and even artificial additives, these two glands work hard to make sure you will not get ill from toxicity, but when they are overworked, you can run into problems.

Detox Tea

1 tsp Milk thistle seeds
(excellent for detoxing the liver)
1 tsp Dandelion root
(good for liver and water retention)

Prostate

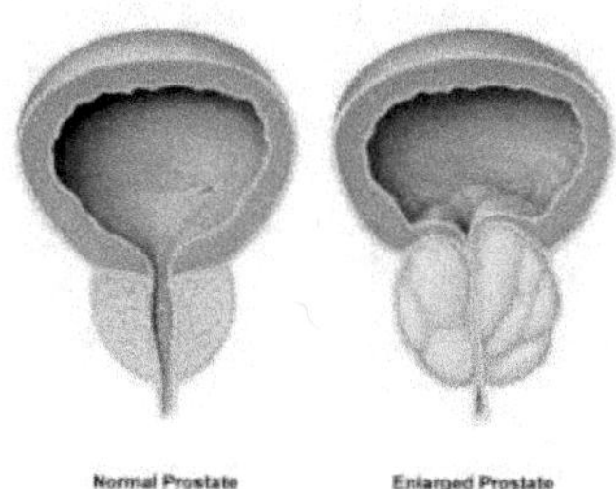

Normal Prostate   Enlarged Prostate

Prostate health is very important for men. Regular checks can lead to early detection for cancer and other prostate problems. There is also something you can take to maintain prostate health.

Saw Palmetto is the best supplement you take on a regular basis to maintain prostate health.

Conclusion

If someone you are with becomes seriously hurt you may need to assist them by moving them from location to location. Having that said, this means that you need to know the *proper way* to move them. If there are signs of a back injury for example, you need to make sure that the patient is rendered immobile in order to prevent any further injury to the back and neck. If you have someone to help you lift this person, that's great, but if you are by yourself you may just have to improvise.

One easy way to move someone would be to use a large article of clothing such as a bed sheet, or large coat to drag the individual. This is done by wrapping the clothing securely around the person's legs. You can then pull your ailing comrade to safety, it may not be the prettiest or most sophisticated way to render aid, but when all else fails, it will get the job done.

Administering CPR

Standing for "cardiopulmonary resuscitation", the technique called CPR is used to apply manual pressure to a heart that has stopped beating. In order to apply CPR, make sure the patient is on their back, on a flat surface. Now kneel beside the patient, positioning in line with their chest. Now place your index finger at the bottom notch of the person's ribs.

Position your hand's heel above this notch. Now place the palm of your hand on top of the other positioned above the notch. Now you can begin your chest compressions. Use a compression rate of 80 to 100 per minute, and stop every 15 to breathe 2 breaths into the person's lungs in between compressions. This emergency prep could be invaluable during a crisis.

Applying a Tourniquet

It's a gruesome reality, but if someone is injured severely enough, they can bleed to death. In order to prevent a tragedy like this, you need to know how to apply a tourniquet. Tourniquet's can be self-applied or applied to others, and simply consist of a material being wrapped around a limb in order to apply pressure and stem the flow of bleeding.

You can make a simple tourniquet simply by ripping a strip of cloth off of your shirt and tying it tightly around the affected area. Make sure the material is at least an inch and a half wide to make sure that it doesn't break and will remain stable. Keep this tourniquet on until you can stabilize the patient.

Giving Heimlich maneuver

If you see someone with a look of clear distress, with their face contorted in fear, unable to speak, unable to even breathe, and they are pointing to their throat, you can be sure that they are choking. In such a desperate situation the Heimlich maneuver is just what the survival doctor ordered. In order to properly administer this life saving maneuver, you need to stand directly behind the choking victim and place your arms around their stomach as if you are giving them a hug.

Now ball your hand into a fist and grab the outside of this fist with your other hand. Now with your elbows pointed out behind you begin energetically thrusting that fist up into the person's stomach causing the wind to shoot up through their diaphragm. This will eventually cause whatever is obstructing their windpipe to shoot out of their mouth. This bit of survival medicine really could save someone's life.

ESSENTIAL OILS
FOR KIDS

GLADYS BEASLEY

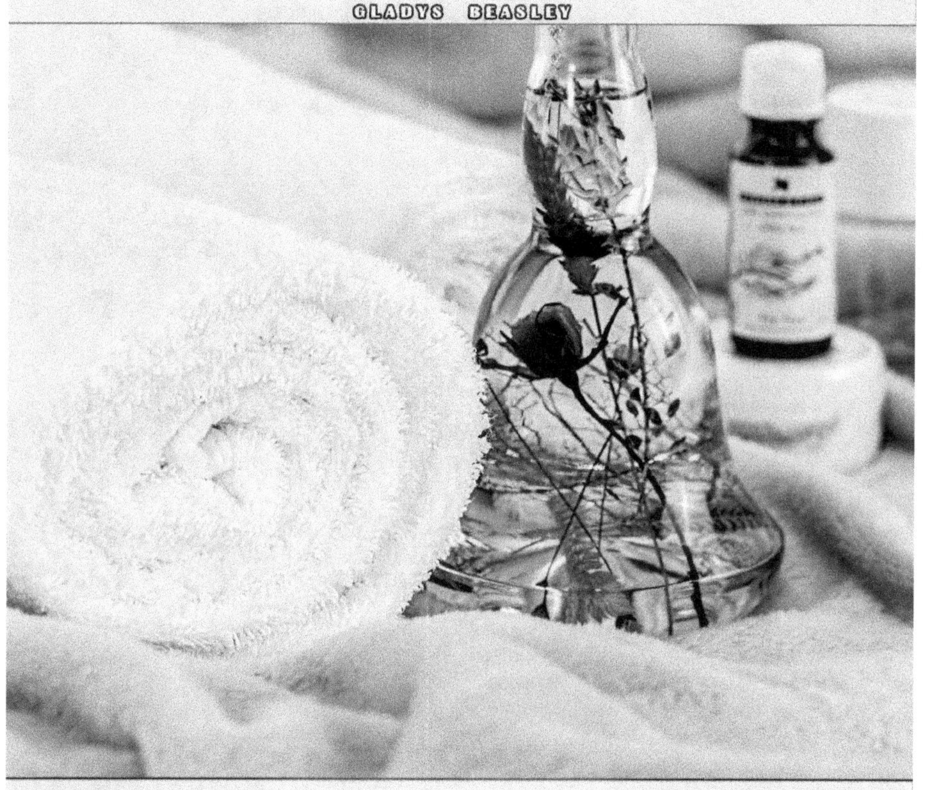

34 DIY NATURAL, TOXIC-FREE RECIPES FOR YOUR CHILDREN'S HEALTH

Essential Oils for Kids:

34 DIY Natural Toxic-Free Recipes For Your Children's Health

Introduction

You're looking for a better way to care for your kids...

You take them to the doctor, give them the best of meals, and make sure nothing happens to them within your power. The problem is you're getting disillusioned with prescription drugs, additives in food, and other chemicals in what they drink, you are looking for a better way to maintain their health to reduce the number of times you have to take them to the doctor for health or other problems.

You've looked online and even talked to a few people who sell essential oils, but all the information is either too much to digest or it seems to contradict itself. Look no further, this book was written with 20+ years experience in the natural health and aromatherapy fields. I will give you all the advice you need to get started with essential oils, and aromatherapy, and helping you to raise your children in a toxic-free environment.

Chapter 1 - Aromatherapy for Kids 101

There are over 90 essential oils on the market, and all of them are used for all sorts of health benefits, but not all are appropriate for children. Different age groups can only use certain essential oils. Out of the over 90 essential oils, there are less than 30 essential oils that are safe for use for children.

Aromatherapy Preparations

From simple blends to soaps and shampoos, there are a lot of ways you can prepare essential oils. Here is a list of them you can do at home:

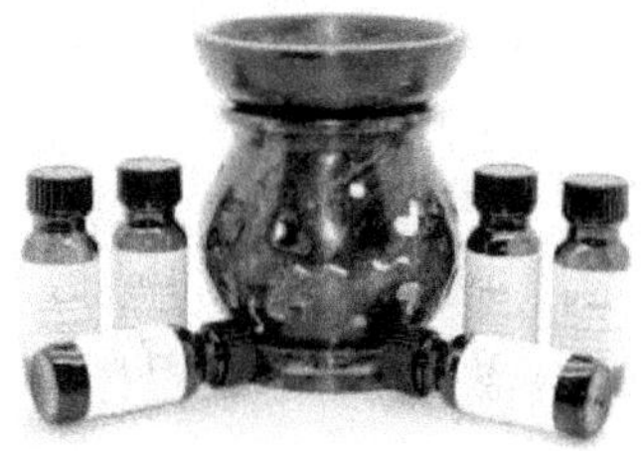

1. Simple Diffuser Blend

This is mixing different essential oils together and placing the mixture either in a diffuser or on a candle warmer.

2. Bath/Mineral Salts

This is a combination of epsom and sea salts with borax and baking soda or ground oatmeal with essential oils and carrier oils. You add it to a bath for different health reasons.

3. Shampoo

You add either add essential oils to an existing shampoo or make your own shampoo from home and control what goes into your shampoo.

4. Soaps

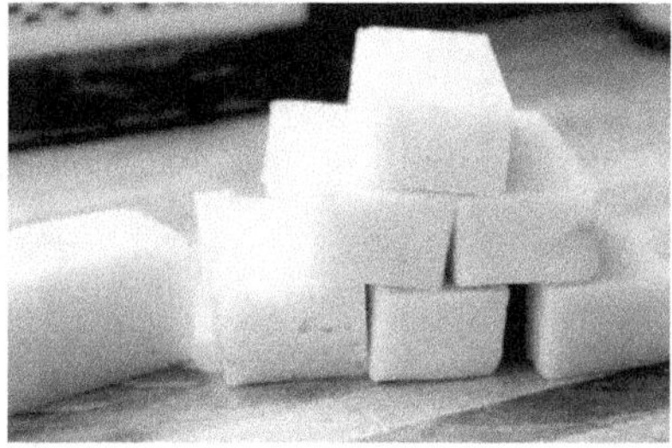

There are melt and pour soaps you can make yourself and add essential oils to.

5. Room Sprays

These are very simply essential blends that have been added to water in a spray bottle to freshen a room or sanitize an area.

6. Massage Oils

These oils can be used as chest rubs and other things for children.

7. Salves and ointments

These are aromatherapy products made from petroleum jelly or bees wax. It will help to keep the essential oils on the area you are trying to treat longer.

Tools of the Trade

Like most hobbies, you need the proper tools to do a proper job, and aromatherapy is no different. Here is a list of tools you will need to make the preparations, and most are already in your kitchen.

Glass Double Boiler

This will come in handy when making salves and ointments. You can also make your own double boiler by placing a glass bowl in a small pot that has boiling water.

Crock Pot

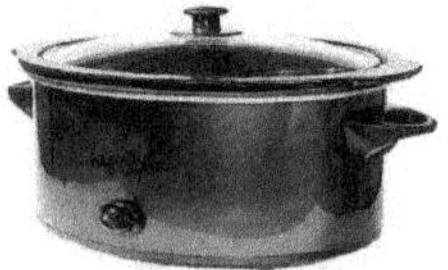

When your making melt and pour soap, you need something to melt in that is bigger than a double boiler. That's where a crock pot comes into play.

Soap Molds

You can find these in any craft shop as well as online. They range from loaf shapes to more artistic molds so you can be creative.

Empty Shampoo Bottles

These can be bottles that you have emptied and cleaned. This will save you a little bit of money.

Air-Tight Containers

They come in all shapes and sizes and you can find them online. They will be a life-saver when making salves and ointments. You can also use them to store your bath and mineral salts.

Measuring cups/spoons

These will help you measure out all the ingredients you will need to make the preparations.

Food Scale

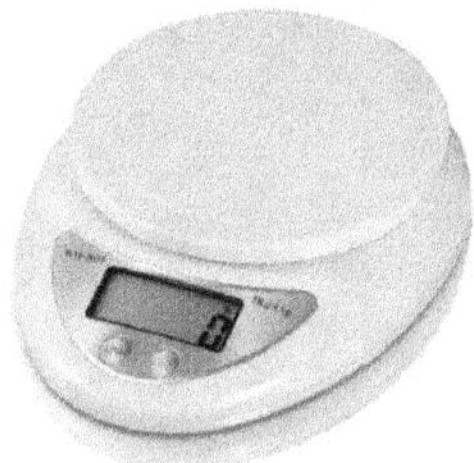

This is for weighing and measuring your dry ingredients like the baking soda and blocks of melt and pour soap.

Spray Bottles

These are for mixing the sanitizing sprays and room sprays.

Wooden Spoons

These are recommend to mix the ingredients when making soaps, ointments, and salves. You can even use silicone mixing tools, if you like.

Blender/Food Processor

This is to mix the shampoos, dry goods and other ingredients together.

Gloves

You need to use these to mix the essential oils. Essential oils can cause contact dermatitis when used undiluted.

Baking Soda

This is a common ingredient in bath salts and mineral baths.

Borax

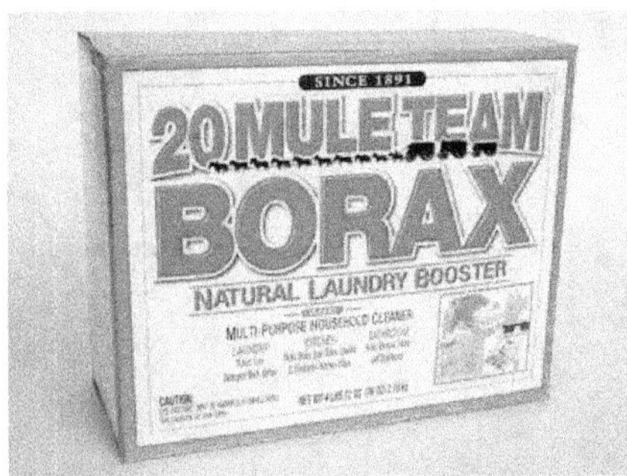

This is a naturally occurring mineral that helps to smooth the skin.

Epsom Salts

This is one of the two salts used in a mineral or bath salts.

Ground Oatmeal

This is usually steel cut oats that have been ground into a fine powder for use in baths. It's used in place of salts in cases of high blood pressure.

Melt and Pour Soap

This can be found in any craft shop or online. It comes in bricks that are graded so you can cut them in ounce increments.

Carrier Oils

These are oils you add essential oils to in order to dilute them.

Labels

It's always good to label your products and date them. Many preparations lose their punch after a certain amount of time and others have to be used immediately.

Salves have a shelf life of 6 months.

Ointments have a shelf life of up to a year.

Shampoos have a shelf life of four months.

Melt and Pour Soaps have a shelf life of up to a year.

Safety First

There are a few things you need to keep in mind when using essential oils:

1. Store in a cool dry place

Essential oils have a habit of evaporating in high temperatures. To avoid this, store your essential oils in a cool dry place, like a pantry.

2. Keep undiluted essential oils out of little ones' reach

Essential oils are toxic undiluted and can cause health issues.

3. Clean your tools before and after use.

This will prevent cross-contamination. You can buy tools just for making the preparations, but since you're not dealing with really caustic materials, it isn't really necessary.

4. Do not ingest essential oils

Some would say this is perfectly safe to do, and I would say only in small doses and mixed into food. It does not matter the grade of essential oil. If it is not diluted, it should not be ingested.

5. Patch Test

This the practice of diluting a small amount of an essential oil and placing it on a small patch of skin to see if you have an adverse reaction to it. This should be performed for all essential oils you are planning on using.

2 drops of essential oil

1 tsp vegetable oil

Mix together and apply a small amount to a patch of skin that is not readily visible. If no reaction is seen within 24 hours, the essential oil is safe to use.

6. Do not use undiluted essential oils on the skin.

Some companies would have you believe this is perfectly fine if they are therapeutic grade essential oils. This is simply not true. Even Lavender, an essential oil commonly used undiluted, can cause contact dermatitis when used too often undiluted.

7. Do not put on infant hands and feet

There are sites out there that say this is a good idea due to the nerves in the hands and feet, and it is, but babies have a tendency of putting their feet and hands in their mouths. So, it's best not to do it.

8. Know where your essential oil is coming from.

Vet the manufacturer and look at how they are rated in terms of purity and how the screen their essential oils. There are companies out there that will try to substitute one essential for another or dilute the oil and not advertise it is diluted.

As you can see, I'm already debunking some information that is out there. Now, let's get on to the rest of the book, starting with the immune system.

Chapter 2 - Essential Oil List

As I mentioned in the previous chapter, not all essential oils are suitable for children under twelve. Here is a list of essential oils and the age groups most appropriate for them. Starting with newborn, you can add the essential oils to the list for the other age groups, but you can not add them in regression.

For instance you can add the newborn essential oils to the 2-12 month list, but you cannot add the 2-12 month list to the newborn essential oil list.

Newborn *Dill (Anethum graveolens)*

This essential oil is good for colic, flatulence, and indigestion

Lavender (Lavandula angustufolia)

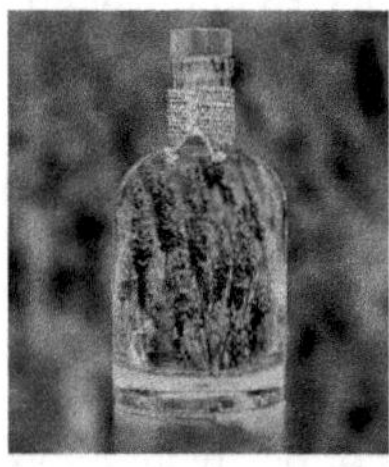

Lavender is the most versatile of the essential oils. You can combine it with virtually every other oil in the market; you can use undiluted sparingly without side effects, and it can be used for a multitude of health reasons:

Dermatitis, earache, eczema, psoriasis, sunburn muscle aches, asthma, bronchitis, whooping cough, colic, flatulence, nausea, flu, insomnia, headache, nervous tension, and dry scalp. That is just the short list.

Roman Chamomile (Chamaemelum nobile)

Highly recommended for sensitive skin, this essential oil has a long list of benefits as well:

Acne, allergies, dermatitis, earache, eczema, insect bites, rashes, nausea, indigestion, colic, insomnia, and nervous tension to name a few.

Yarrow (Achillea millefolium)

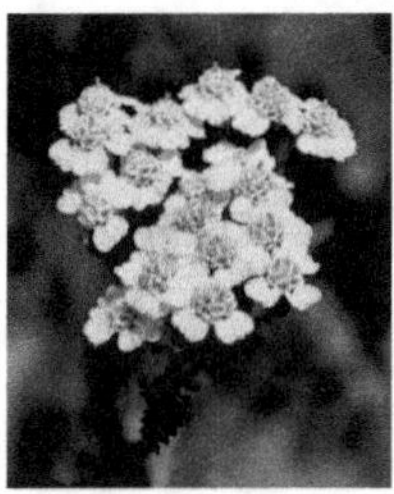

This essential oil is not as famous as the two above it, but it does come in handy for helping with acne, the treatment of burns, eczema, rashes, lessening scars, toning the skin, cramps, flatulence, indigestion, colds, breaking fevers, flu, insomnia, an is often added to hair rinses.

2-12 Months

Geranium (Pelargonium graveolens)

This floral oil has been used in the treatment of bruises, burns, congested skin, dermatitis, eczema, oily complexions, tonsillitis, sore throats, and nervous tension. *Can cause dermatitis in highly sensitive skin.*

Tangerine/Mandarin (Citrus reticulata)

This essential oil is labeled as one or the other in most natural health stores and online. This is why I include the Latin name of the oil. This oil is known to help with congested and oily skin, lightening of scars, a skin toner, intestinal problems, digestive problems, insomnia, nervous tension, and restlessness.

Eucalyptus (Eucalyptus globulus)

Well known for being used in vaporizers and other diffusion devices, eucalyptus has been used to open nasal passages and congested chests. It can also help treat insect bites, skin infections, ease muscular aches and pains, sprains, and throat infections. It is also effective in treating bronchitis, sinusitis, colds, flu, and measles.

Tea Tree (Melaleuca alternifolia)

This essential oil is the perfect substitute for use in killing mold, mildew and bacteria. It is also used to treat acne, athlete's foot, burns, cold sores, dandruff, insect bites, oily skin, rashes, asthma, bronchitis, coughs, sinusitis, whooping cough, thrush, colds, fever, flu, chicken pox, measles.

12 Months-5 Years

Palmarosa (Cymnopogon martinii)

This essential oil has been known to help with acne, dermatitis, minor skin infections, scarring, facials, oily skin, dry skin, intestinal infections.

5 Years - 12 Years

Clary Sage (Salvia sclarea)

This is another strong essential oil, but it's good for use in this age rage. Since it is a little more potent than the ones before it, I would not recommend making it the mainstay of a blend. Two to three drops should be enough for a tablespoon. This oil is good to help with acne, dandruff, oily skin and hair, muscular aches and pains, intestinal cramps and flatulence.

Nutmeg (Myristica fragrans)

This aromatic oil is used for helping treat muscular aches and pains, flatulence, indigestion, nausea, and bacterial infections. *This essential oil is toxic in large doses.*

Chapter 3 - The Immune System

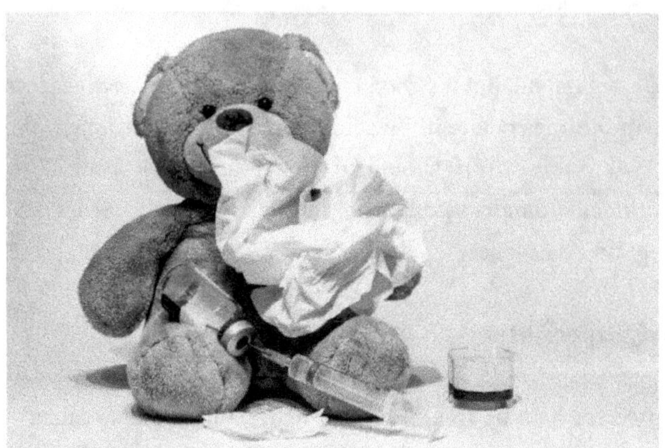

This is the system that fights infections, colds, the flu and other diseases. In today's world it's unheard of to let our children play outside barefoot, drink out of water hoses, and even just get muddy for fear of germs, but did you know depriving them of that actually isn't good for their immune system?

Your body is constantly exposed to a germ-filled environment on a daily basis. This allows your immune system to adapt to the bombardment and become stronger. This is the same for your children. We want to provide a sterile environment for them, but that does not allow their immune systems to become as strong as they need to be to cope with everyday bacteria and germs.

There are some things you can do to help their immune system prevent them from getting sick:

1. They need plenty of sleep

Toddlers 1-3 years: 11-14 hours of sleep
Preschoolers 3-5 years: 10-13 hours of sleep
6-13 years: 9-11 hours

This may seem like a lot, but they are still developing their immune systems, and they need all the rest they can get. This is why it is recommended toddlers to 5 years of age need to take naps.

2. Balanced diet

Fruits, vegetables, meats, grains, fats, and the rest of the pyramid in a proper balance is essential to the development of a growing child and their immune system. When you start them early on healthy snacks, they will carry that habit with them as they grow.

3. Let them play

Between day care or school, chores, and homework, there is one thing that can get lost in the shuffle at times, play. They need to go outside and play, whether it be on a bicycle or in-line skates, playing a sport, or just pretending they're Jedi or superheroes, children need to play. It's good their immune system and their imagination.

4. Spending time with them

Your children need you to spend quality time with them. This time can mean watching shows with them, playing catch, or even reading them a bedtime story. They need their parents to interact with them to form bonds, and be reassured they are loved. It's one thing to a child to be told they are loved.

Chest Rub

When your child's chest is congested, you want to do anything you can to alleviate the coughing and hacking. Here are a couple of recipes you can use to help them breathe and sleep better.

Newborn Chest Rub

1/2 Cup Coconut oil

1 tbsp beeswax pastilles (Little beads)

2 tbsp Shea butter

5 Drops Lavender essential oil

5 Drops Yarrow Essential oil

- In a double boiler, place the coconut oil, beeswax, and Shea Butter.
- Mix the essential oils and set aside
- Stir until it is melted.
- Place in a tightly lidded container.
- When it is still warm and not hot, stir in the essential oils
- To use, spread a light layer on the chest.

12 Months to 5 Years Chest Rub

1/2 Cup Coconut oil

1 tbsp beeswax pastilles (Little beads)

2 tbsp Shea butter

5 Drops Eucalyptus Essential oil

5 Drops Mandarin Essential oil

5 Drops Geranium Essential oil

- In a double boiler, place the coconut oil, beeswax, and Shea Butter.
- Mix the essential oils and set aside
- Stir until it is melted.
- Place in a tightly lidded container.
- When it is still warm and not hot, stir in the essential oils
- To use, spread a light layer on the chest.

Fevers

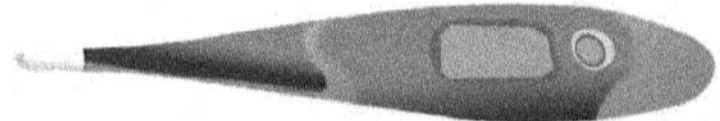

Nothing stops us in our tracks faster than kissing our child on the forehead and feeling it is hot to the touch. Our first instinct is always to call the doctor and then reach for something to break the fever. A fever is the immune system's way of fighting off the infection by burning it out of the system. I am not saying to let the fever rage. I saying it is better to regulate the fever instead of trying to keep it down until it breaks. This will give the body a fighting chance to get rid of the infection that is inside the body trying to take hold.

There is one circumstance in which you need to need to go to the emergency room when your child has a fever:

When the fever is in a steady increase no matter what you have done to regulate it, and it's been constantly rising for the course of the day.

Here are the limits of the temperatures of your child and when you need to take them to the doctor:

3-6 mos. 101F
Over 6 mos: 103F+
Any age: 104F+

You can control the temperature of the child by placing them in a bath that matches their body temperature at the time and then slowly introducing cool water to lower the water temperature.

Do not place a child with a fever in an ice bath.

Their system will go into shock because of the extreme temperature change.

2-12 Month Fever Bath

1 Cup Epsom Salts
1/4 Cup Sea Salt
1/4 Cup Baking Soda
5 drops Yarrow Essential Oil
5 Drops Tea Tree Essential Oil
3 Tbsp Sweet Almond Oil

- Mix the dry ingredients and set aside
- Mix the oils together and add to the dry ingredients
- Place in container with a tight lid overnight
- Place an 1/8 cup of the salts in running water and mix well.

12 Months -5 Years Fever Bath

1 Cup Epsom Salts
1/4 Cup Sea Salt
1/4 Cup Baking Soda
5 drops Eucalyptus Essential Oil
5 Drops Tea Tree Essential Oil
5 Drops Lavender Essential Oil
3 Tbsp Sweet Almond Oil

- Mix the dry ingredients and set aside
- Mix the oils together and add to the dry ingredients
- Place in container with a tight lid overnight
- Place an 1/8 cup of the salts in running water and mix well.

Room Diffusers

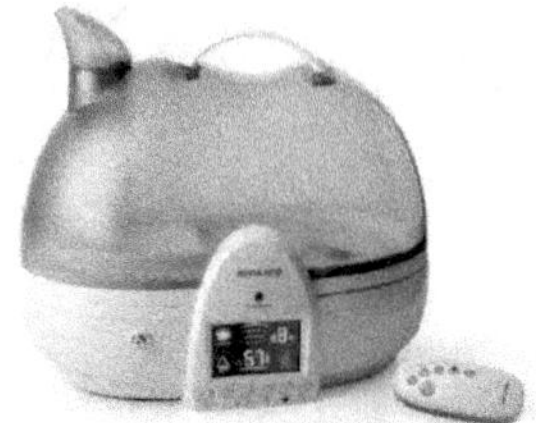

Sometimes it is best to have diffuser blends. These blends are placed either in a diffuser or a candle warmer. The release of the aroma of the blend will be inhaled as it travels through the air.

Newborn Immune Booster Blend

5 Drops Roman Chamomile Essential Oil

3 Drops Lavender Essential Oil

2 Drops Yarrow Essential Oil

1/4 cup Filtered Water

- Mix all ingredients well and place in diffuser
- Leave out the water and place 5 drops on a candle warmer

5-12 Year Immune Booster Blend

5 Drops Lavender Essential Oil

3 Drops Clary Sage Essential Oil

2 Drops Nutmeg Essential Oil

1/4 cup Filtered Water

- Mix all ingredients well and place in diffuser
- Leave out the water and place 5 drops on a candle warmer.

Chapter 4 - Dry Skin

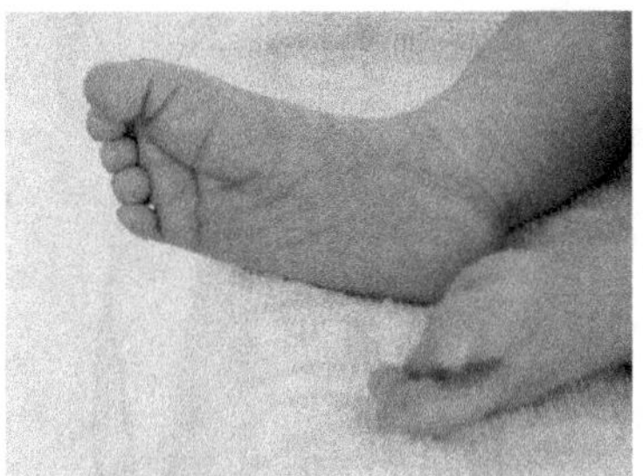

The dry patches, redness, and irritation that comes along with dry skin can be frustrating to us, but can you imagine how bad it can be to your child, especially when you tell them *not* to scratch the rash? Rashes can be due to poison ivy or some allergic reaction to something either ingested or that touched the skin. Rashes can be as simple as a small reddish patch on the skin to more severe cases like eczema or psoriasis. The good news they are treatable and avoidable if they are allergic reactions. To find out if your child has any allergies, you can take them to their pediatrician and ask for an allergen test.

Rashes can also be caused by stress and nervousness. If your child gets anxious when they have to speak in from of a class or large group of people or even be introduced to new people, they can develop a anxiety related skin condition. There is always a reason for the rash, and often that reason is a simple one.

Bathing in lukewarm or cool water will help the skin retain moisture while hot water will dry it out. Think about it for a minute. When you boil water, the meat shrinks as does any vegetable you boil in it. The same concept applies to your skin. It will wrinkle and not have the same elastic quality it should, making it easy to get cuts and rashes.

Lotions

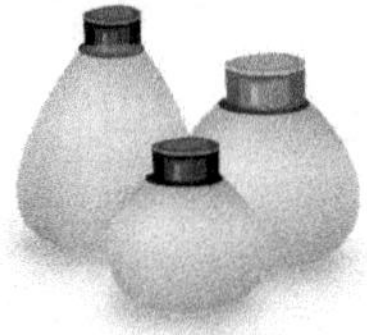

You can purchase the lotion base already made to save you the trouble. You can find it in hobby shops and online. You will also need a bottle to store the lotion. Here are a couple of lotion recipes you can use for your little one.

Newborn Rash Cream

2 ounces of lotion base

10 Drops Lavender Essential Oil

5 Drops Roman Chamomile Essential Oil

Mix all the ingredients together using a hand mixer and pour into the container. Place a small amount on the rash. If using on diaper rash, avoid the genital area.

12 Month to 5 Years Poison Ivy Cream

2 ounces of lotion base

10 Drops Palmarosa Essential Oil

5 Drops Roman Chamomile Essential Oil

5 Drops Tea Tree Essential Oil

Mix all the ingredients together using a hand mixer and pour into the container. Place a small amount on the rash. If using on diaper rash, avoid the genital area.

Body Butters

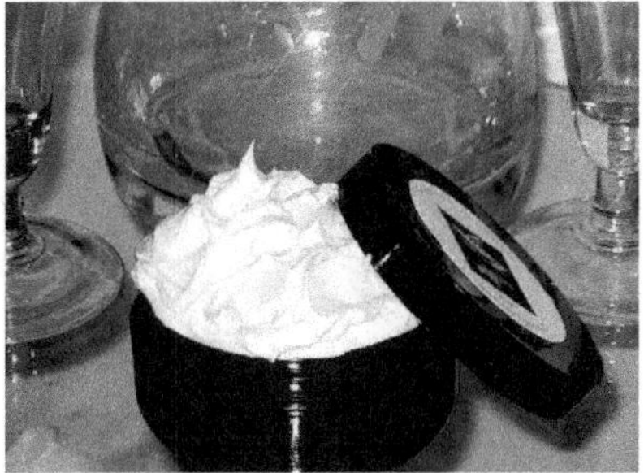

These are often found at stores in short, round containers and come in avocado, shea and other butters. Much like the lotion base, you can also find them online. You can also mix them together to increase effectiveness. You can make lotions for eczema or psoriasis, but body butters will last longer on the skin allowing the essential oils to stay on the area longer. You can also prevent the butter from rubbing off by having them wear a glove or wrapping the area with a bandage.

2-12 Months Eczema/Psoriasis

1 Ounce Avocado Butter
1 Ounce Shea Butter
10 Drops Geranium Essential Oil
5 Drops Roman Chamomile Essential Oil
5 Drops Yarrow Essential Oil

- Mix the Butters and set aside
- Mix the essential oils and set aside
- Using a hand mixer, blend the essential oils into the butters
- Place the butter in an air-tight container

5-12 Years Eczema/Psoriasis

1 Ounce Avocado Butter

1 Ounce Shea Butter

10 Drops Palmarosa Essential Oil

5 Drops Tea Tree Essential Oil

5 Drops Lavender Essential Oil

5 Drops Roman Chamomile Essential Oil

- Mix the Butters and set aside
- Mix the essential oils and set aside
- Using a hand mixer, blend the essential oils into the butters
- Place the butter in an air-tight container

All-Purpose Lotion

These two lotions can be used on an everyday basis for those days the skin looks a little ashy or for out of the bath.

Newborn

2 Ounces Lotion Base
15 Drops Lavender Essential Oil

Mix them together well. You can use this before putting your newborn to bed to help them sleep.

2-12 Months

2 Ounces Lotion Base
5 Drops Tangerine/Mandarin Essential Oil
5 Drops Geranium Essential Oil
5 Drops Roman Chamomile Essential Oil

Chapter 5 - Homework and Concentration

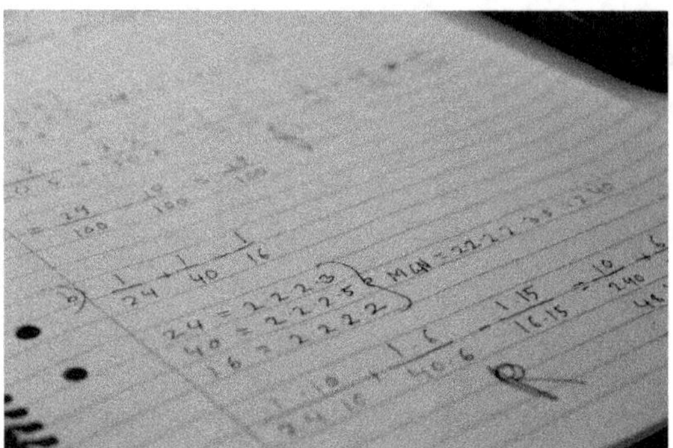

The hardest thing to do sometimes is getting your children to sit long enough to do their homework. They fidget, they squirm, and their focus tends to wane. Here are some things you can do to help them concentrate better.

1. Let them blow off some steam

Their fresh from having to sit for a few hours before they come home, and then there is the ride home, whether bus or car. Let them play for a bit before starting their homework. This lets them expend any extra energy, and they will fidget less. The best time for them to do their homework is normally after dinner.

2. Sit with them

Help them do their homework or just sit with them as they do it. You can read a book, write in a journal or anything else you can think of, but sitting with them as they do their homework will let them know you are there if they happen to get stuck.

3. No distractions

Turn the Television off and confiscate their phone and other electronic devices. All these serve to distract them from getting their work done. If they need a calculator, by them a simple one or one suited to help them do the math they are currently practicing. If they want music, play jazz or classical. Soothing tones can help keep energy evened out and their mind on the task at hand.

These blends are focused on leveling out energy and toning down fidgeting. These are all diffuser blends for children 12 months to 12 Years.

Concentration Blend I

5 Drops Lavender Essential Oil
5 Drops Tangerine/Mandarin Essential Oil

Concentration Blend II

5 Drops Roman Chamomile Essential Oil
5 Drops Tangerine/Mandarin Essential Oil

ADD/ADHD

They act out, come home with endless notes on behavior and can't seem to sit still for anything, and you have tried everything short of tying them to a chair. You're at the end of your rope, and so you take your child to the doctor, and after a battery of testing, they tell you your child has either ADD or ADHD. It's not the end of the world. You now know the problem. Here are some things you can do help them.

1. Reduce sugars and artificial additives in the diet

This may seem like an insurmountable task, but switching to an all natural diet will help immensely. Don't know how to start? Feingold.org can help with that. Feingold is a doctor that was able to prove many learning disabilities stem from a diet laden with artificial preservatives, flavors, and colors. The website can walk you through the steps on living a life free of those.

2. Give them a little caffeine.

Hear me out. When you give caffeine to a hyper child, they slow down and calm down. I know it sounds incredulous, but it's true. Caffeine acts like a depressant in the systems of those who suffer from ADD and ADHD.

Peppermint (Mentha Piperita)

I am introducing this essential oil here because it does help with concentration and nervous tension. I have used several times when I have needed to stay on task.
The following blends are for ages 5 years and up.

ADD Blend I

5 Drops Peppermint Essential Oil
5 Drops Lavender Essential Oil

Blend well and either put five drops on a candle warmer or follow the directions for a diffuser.

ADD Blend II

3 Drops Peppermint Essential Oil
2 Drops Geranium Essential Oil
5 Drops Tangerine/Mandarin Essential Oil

Chapter 6 - Bedtime and Nervousness

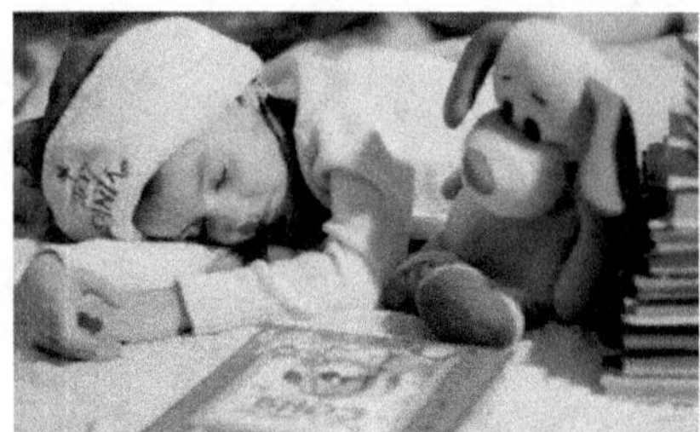

All of us who are parents know one simple truth about children. It's a battle to get them to go to bed. They don't want to miss anything and will *do* anything to stay up "Just a little bit longer". From asking for one more story to wanting to watch TV with you, there is no end to the negotiation at bedtime. Here are a couple of recipes you can use to help them drift off to sleep.

Hyperactivity Blend I

5 drops Chamomile Essential Oil
5 Drops Geranium Essential Oil
In a diffuser or candle warmer.

Hyperactivity Blend II

5 Drops Tangerine/Mandarin Essential Oil
5 Drops Chamomile Essential Oil

Whether it's the night before a big test or right before a recital or game, kids are a bundle of nerves and nervous energy. Here are a couple of recipes to help them calm down before those events.

Nervous Blend I

2 Drops Clary Sage Essential Oil

3 Drops Pepperminy Essential Oil

5 Drops Tangerine/Mandarin Essential Oil

Nervous Blend II

3 Drops Lavender Essential Oil

3 Drops Tangerine Essential Oil

2 Drops Geranium Essential Oil

2 Drops Clary Sage Essential Oil

Sleep Aid I

5 Drops Yarrow Essential Oil

3 Drops Chamomile Essential Oil

2 Drops Tangerine/Mandarin Essential Oil

Sleep Aid II

3 Drops Geranium Essential Oil

3 Drops Peppermint Essential Oil

4 Drops Yarrow Essential Oil

Chapter 7 - Bath Time

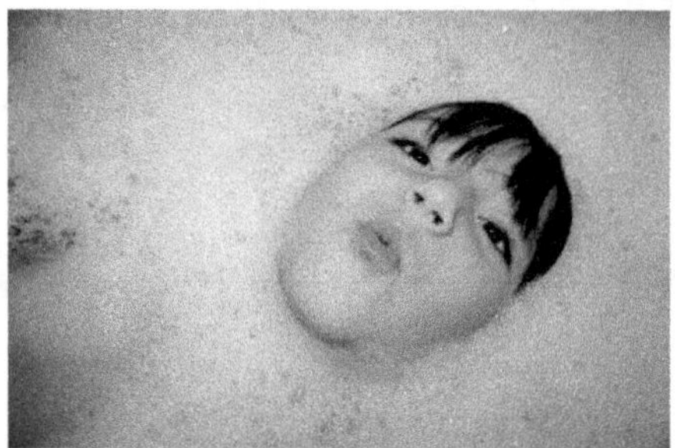

Kids get dirty. We can dress them up and they seem to attract dirt in a matter of seconds. Finding the right products to keep them clean without tons of chemicals is tricky. You can buy plain shampoo base from health retailers online.

Shampoo for Oily hair 5 Years+

4 Ounces Shampoo base
10 Drops Geranium Essential Oil
10 Drops Tangerine/Mandarin Essential Oil

Mix well and use as normal.

Shampoo 2-12 Months Oily Hair

2 Ounces Shampoo base
10 Drops Geranium Oil
5 Drops Lavender Essential Oil

Mix well and use as normal.

Dry Shampoo 2-12 mos

2 Ounces Shampoo base
10 Drops Chamomile Essential Oil
5 Drops Lavender Essential Oil

Lice

The ban of every parent of school age children, lice are insidious. They get everywhere if not treated.

Lice Shampoo I 5 years+

4 Ounces Shampoo base
10 Drops Palmarosa Essential Oil
10 Drops Tea Tree Essential Oil
5 Drops Clary Sage Essential Oil

Lice Shampoo II 5 years+

4 Ounces Shampoo base
10 Drops Lavender Essential Oil
10 Drops Tangerine/Mandarin Essential Oil
5 Drops Tea Tree Oil Essential Oil

Body Soap for newborns

4 Ounces Goat's Milk Melt and Pour Soap
15 Drops Lavender Essential Oil

- Melt the soap in a double boiler
- Pour the soap in a mold
- Add the essential oil in when the soap is warm and you can still stir it

Soap for Boys 5+

4 Ounces Olive Oil Melt and Pour Soap

10 Drops Tangerine/Mandarin Essential Oil

10 Drops Palmarosa Essential Oil

5 Drops Clary Sage Essential Oil

Girls' Soap ages 5 and up Dry Skin

4 Ounces Goat's Milk Melt and Pour Soap

10 Drops Lavender Essential Oil

10 Drops Peppermint Essential Oil

5 Drops Palmarosa Essential Oil

- Mix the essential oils before you add them to the soap.

Girls' Soap ages 5 and up Oily Skin

4 Ounces Goat's Milk Melt and pour Soap

10 Drops Tangerine/Mandarin Essential Oil

10 Drops Geranium Essential Oil

5 Drops Palmarosa Essential Oil

- Mix the essential oils before you add them to the soap.

Facial Care

As they get older, kids need a different soap to cleanse their faces. Here are a few recipes you can use. All of these are for children ages 5 and up.

Recipe I (for pimples)

4 Ounces Olive Oil Melt and Pour

5 Drops Eucalyptus Essential Oil

10 Drops Palmarosa Essential oil

5 Drops Tea Tree Essential Oil

5 Drops Lavender Essential Oil

Recipe II (Oily Skin)

4 Ounces Goat's Milk Melt and Pour Soap

10 Drops Tangerine/Mandarin Essential Oil

10 Drops Geranium Essential Oil

5 Drops Clary Sage Essential Oil

Recipe III (Dry Skin)

4 Ounces Goat's Milk Melt and Pour Soap

10 Drops Lavender Essential Oil

10 Drops Chamomile Essential Oil

5 Drops Yarrow Essential Oil

Chapter 8 - Tips and Tricks

Here is a list of quick things you can do when you don't have all of the ingredients to make the recipes.

1.   You can add 3 drops to every tablespoon of shampoo to help treat lice.

2.   You can add 3 drops of Lavender essential oils to every tablespoon of liquid soap to sooth your infant's nerves before bed. This will help them sleep.

3.   To help speed healing in cases of sunburn, add 3 drops of Lavender to each tablespoon of Aloe gel.

4.   Three drops of Eucalyptus on your child's night light before plugging it in will help them breathe better when they have a cold.

It doesn't stop there

You can find forums online to help further your knowledge of essential oils and aromatherapy. You can find new recipes, get advice, and even suggest some of your own. There is no end to the learning.

Conclusion

I hope the information in this book has helped get you started in your new and rewarding facet of natural health. There are myriads of books and sites you can use to continue your education. Until next time, stay well.

www.ingramcontent.com/pod-product-compliance
Lightning Source LLC
Chambersburg PA
CBHW071023260726
48662CB00024B/1782